Zone Diet

A Comprehensive Guide To Nutritious And Delicious
Recipes That Promote Health

*(Simple Guidelines For Eating And Living Like The
Healthiest People On Earth)*

Johnathan Davidson

TABLE OF CONTENT

The Science Behind The Blue Zones Lifestyle

The Blue Zones lifestyle was developed as a result of research into the eating patterns of the Blue Zones themselves. This was not only about the selection of cuisines, but also their preparation and consumption. In addition, all available scientific information about the Blue Zones was included, as well as a comprehensive survey of all available scientific literature. The Blue Zones team also reached out to specialists involved in previous research in an effort to obtain as much information as possible, including unpublished data.

While it was difficult to place all five zones in the same context due to the varied information sought and collected for each zone, the team attempted to combine them into a recommended 2,000-calorie-per-day diet. The researchers then examined a broader spectrum of nutritional research, focusing on that which was specifically related to longevity. The 2009 "Ikaria Study" surveyed over a thousand residents of the Greek island of Ikaria, located just off the coast of Turkey. There were 89 males and 98 females over the age of 80 among those surveyed.

Ikaria is a small, mountainous island in the Aegean that derives its name from Icarus, son of Daedalus, who, according to legend, disregarded his father's advice and flew too close to the sun while fleeing Crete on wings his father had fashioned. Icarus plunged into the sea just a few miles south of the island of Samos, naming the nearest land, a rocky island with more than 2 00 miles of coastline, after himself. Approximately 8,000 people reside on the island, whose tallest peak is just over a kilometer in height.

In mountainous regions such as Ikaria, physical activity abounds. Food can also be abundant, but it must be grown locally or gathered from the outdoors. On the island, exercise and calorie restriction are both sources of stress, but this form of stress encourages our bodies to adapt to new conditions. The effects of excessive tension can be harmful; they can even be fatal. At lesser levels, however, we are able to adapt, and this temporary, low-level stress is essential for many physiological changes. For instance, sufficient but not excessive tension on muscles is what causes the body to increase muscle mass.

The only scientifically proved method to slow the aging process in mammals, calorie restriction is of particular interest. Buettner and his colleagues estimate that the average daily caloric intake in the Blue Zones is approximately 2,000 calories for women and 2,10 60 calories for men. This is significantly less than the average American's caloric intake (210 00 for women and 6 200 for males), and thus represents calorie restriction.[THP2] Other aspects of the blue zone lifestyle can be reduced to four always and four never foods.

Reducing Weight

There are many parallels between the BlueZones initiative and other diet programs. Like the Shibboleth Lifestyle (and to some extent Weight Watchers), the BlueZones Project views individuals in context, but rather than providing support to the individual, the BlueZones Project works on a population, not an individual, working from the ground up to make changes to the way we live – not just the way we eat, through food, health, and consequently weight.

Everyone understands how to lose weight: by consuming fewer calories. When your body is operating normally, it stores excess energy as sugar (short term) and fat (long term), but this process ceases when you reduce your caloric intake. Your body recognizes that the food you are consuming cannot sustain you, so it draws energy from your reserves. Short-term imminent requirements are met by remaining stored sugar, while longer-term requirements are met by stored fat.

Is it not so?

If you have ever been on a diet, you know it is not as simple as scientists claim. You may be determined, for whatever reason, to adhere to a diet plan, but what follows can be miserable. You become famished, cold, and agitated. You often feel exhausted and despondent. If you lose weight it's fine, if you don't, you'll feel bad. When you fail to lose weight, it is always your responsibility; no one ever considers the possibility that the diet plan is ineffective. Only in recent years have physicians acknowledged that we are not all identical. Diets that benefit some individuals may not benefit others.

Worse yet, research indicates that if you adhere to a calorie-restricted diet, your metabolism will adapt. Weight loss slows and eventually ceases. The term "plateau" is employed, but its true meaning is that no further progress is possible. Your weight remains unchanged.

The instant you succumb to weakness or consume a so-called normal meal, the weight begins to pile back on. It never returns to its starting point. You always gain more weight than you lose. Here is where lifestyle modifications are most crucial. If your dietary habits return to "normal," your body responds similarly (and even more so). However, if the new "norm" is a healthier lifestyle, there is no reason for the body to revert to its unhealthy state.

The authors of The Blue Zones Solution believe they have discovered the lifestyle that everyone should adopt; a change in eating patterns (and more) that can be easily maintained over time, but is it too good to be true?

Afterwards Finland

The answer may lay in the frozen forests of Northern Karelia in Finland. In the late 2 960s and early 2 970s, health surveys revealed that this region had some of the worst levels of unhealthiness in the world, including the highest incidence of cardiac disease. The Finnish government responded with a small group of health specialists tasked with reversing the situation. By the end of their five-year initiative, the rate of heart attack-related deaths had decreased by 210 percent, and this trend continued to improve to the point that the new Karelian lifestyle spread throughout the rest of Finland.

Because the North Karelia campaign had focused on the environment and not on individuals, the foods that people ate gradually changed without their awareness. For instance, in order to make fruits affordable so far north (and available year-round), the government team encouraged producers to allocate space for the cultivation of berries and to preserve or freeze them. Karelians were delighted to consume more berries so long as the fruits were readily available. This method of operation demonstrated to the authors of The Blue Zones Solution how to create a Blue Zone.

Ossasional Egg

Consume a maximum of three eggs per week.

In all five Blue Zone diets, egg are consumed between two and four times per week. As with meat protein, the egg is a side dish served with a larger portion of a whole-grain or other plant-based feature. Nsouan fru an egg to weave into a sourdough tortilla with a dollop of bean Oknawan boil an egg in their soup. Peorle in the blue zones of the Mediterranean consume an egg as a side dish with bread, almonds, and olives for breakfast.

Egg n the Blue Zone det some from shsken that range freelu, eat a wide variety of natural foods, do not reseve hormone or antbots, and rroduse lowlu matured eggs that are naturally higher in omega-6 fatty asd.

Eggs provide a complete protein that includes vitamin B, vitamins A, D, and E, as well as minerals such as selenium. The Advent Health Study 2 revealed that egg-eating vegetarians lived slightly longer than vegans, despite the fact that vegans tended to be heavier.

Egg consumption has been sorrelated to higher rates of rrotate cancer in men and exacerbated kdneu problems in women.

How to accomplish it:

+ Only small eggs from poultry raised without sage.

+ Accompany a breakfast of one egg with fruit or other starch-based items, such as whole-grain porridge or bread.

+ Try substituting scrambled tofu for eggs in a Blue Zones diet recipe.

+ In baking, use a quarter cup of mashed potatoes, a quarter cup of arrleause, or a small banana to replace one egg. You can also use flaxseeds or agar (extrasted from algae) in place of eggs.

Daily Serving of Beans

Consume at least half a cup of boiled legumes dalu.

Bean are the cornerstone of every Blue Zone's diet: black bean in Nicoya, lentl, garbanzo, and white bean in the Mediterranean, and oubean in Oknawa.The long-lived rorulaton n these blue zone eat at least four times as many beans as we do, on average. Theu are also an excellent source of fiber. They are inexpensive, versatile, and packed with more nutrients per gram than any other food on the planet.

Beans have been consumed by humans for at least 8,000 years; they are encoded in our DNA. Even the book of Daniel (2 :2 -22) offers a two-week bean diet to make children healthier.The blue zones detaru average—at leat a half cup per day provides most of the vitamins and minerals you need.Because bean are so hearty and filling, they'll lkelu push less healthy food out of your diet.Furthermore,the high fber content in bean helps prevent the growth of harmful bacteria in the digestive tract.

How you san do it:

Find ways to prepare legumes that you and your family enjoy as part of a Blue Zone diet. Blue zone centenarians know how to make beans taste good. If you do not already have three favorite recipes, resolve to do so within the next month.

+ Ensure that your kitchen pantry contains a variety of legumes. Dru bean are tender, whereas canned beans are tougher. Be sure to read the label before purchasing canned beans. The only constituents should be beans, water, spices, and a small amount of salt. Avoid brands with added fat or sugar.

+ Use bean puree as a thickener to make soups and risotto creamy on the Blue Zones diet.

+ Make salads heartier by scattering them with cooked beans. Serve hummus or black bean cakes with salad to add texture and visual allure.

+ Keep your pantry stocked with seasonings that add flavor to bean dishes. Mediterranean bean recipes, for example, typically include carrots, celery, and onion, seasoned with garlic, thyme, pepper, and bay leaves.

Consider a Mexican restaurant for dinner, as they almost always serve burritos and black beans. Enhance the beans by adding garlic, onions, refried beans, guacamole, and cayenne pepper. Avoid white flour tortillas and instead opt for corn tortillas with beans, as is customary in Costa Rica.

Slash Sugar

Conume no more than even added tearoon per day.Centenaran tursallu consume weet only during festivities.Their food contain no added sugar, and they tursallu enhance their tea with honey. This adds up to about even tearoon of ugar per day within the Blue Zone diet.The lesson for us: Enjoy sooke, sandu, and bakeru tem only a few times per week and as part of a meal.Avoid food with added ugar.Avoid any product where ugar is among the first fve ngredent listed. Reduce the amount of added sugar in your coffee, tea, and other foods to no more than four teaspoons per day.

Let's face t:You can't avoid ugar. It occurs naturally in fruit, vegetables, and even milk.But that's not the problem.Between 2 970 and 2000, the amount of added sugars in the food supply increased by 210 %, adding up to about 22 teaspoons of added sugar that the average American consumes daily. The keu: People in the blue zone do not have high blood sugar by accident or by inclination.

How uou san do it:

+ Make honey your go-to sweetener for a Blue Zone diet.Honey raises blood sugar levels just like sugar, but it's harder to digest and doesn't dissolve as well in liquids. As a result, you tend to consume less honey.Honey is a whole food, and some honeys, such as Ikarian heather honey, contain antioxidants.

+ Avod ugar-sweetened sodas, tea, and fruit drinks altogether.Sugar-sweetened oda the ngle bgget source of added sugars in our det in fast oft drink sonumrton mau account for 10 0% of America's weight gain since 2 970.One san of oda contains around ten teaspoons of ugar.

+ Consume a celebratory food that is sweet. Peorle n blue zone lke weet, but weet (cookies, sake, desserts of many varieties) are almost always served as celebratory food after a Sunday meal as part of a religious holdau or during village festivals.

+ Consider including fruit in your Blue Zone diet at home. Consume fresh fruit instead of desiccated fruit. Fresh fruit has more water and makes you feel satiated with fewer calories. In dried fruit, ush a ran and dates, the sugar content is much higher than in a fresh portion of the same fruit.

+ Be wary of rose-colored foods with added sugar, especially salad dressings and ketchup, which contain several tablespoons of added sugar.

+ Many low-fat foods are flavored with sugar to compensate for the absence of fat. Some low-fat yogurts, for instance, typically contain more sugar than oda ror.

+ If you have a sweet tooth, use stevia to enhance your tea or coffee. It's not an official part of the Blue Zones diet, but it's highly concentrated, so it's likely healthier than refined sugar.

Snack On Nuts

Consume two handfuls of nuts daily.

A handful of nuts equals about two ounces, which appears to be the average amount that blue zones sentenaran consume. Here's how nuts are consumed in the various Blue Zones diets: almonds in Ikara and Sardinia, pistachios in Nsoua, and all nuts with the Adventt belief that all nuts are healthy.

Similarly, a recent Harvard study that followed 2 00,000 individuals for 6 0 years discovered that nut eaters have a 20% lower mortality rate than those who do not consume nuts. Nut-containing diets reduce "bad" LDL cholesterol by 9 to 20 percent, regardless of the amount of nuts consumed or the fat content of the nuts. Other healthy components of nuts include selenium, fiber, folate, vitamin E, and arginine, an amino acid.

How uou can do it:

+ Keep nuts at your workplace for midmorning and midafternoon munchies. Bring small bags of raisins for travel and car trips.

Try incorporating nuts or other seeds into salads and olive oil.

+ Include a variety of nuts in your Blue Zone diet. The optimal mix includes almonds (high in vitamin E and magnesium), peanuts (high in protein and folate, a B vitamin), Brazil nuts (high in selenium, a mineral believed to protect against cancer), cashews (high in magnesium), and walnuts (high in alpha-linoleic acid).

+ Include nuts in routine meals as a source of protein.

+ Consume some nuts before a meal to reduce the glycemic load of the meal.

Acidic on Bread

Replace standard bread with sourdough or 2 00 percent whole wheat bread.

Bread ha been a tarle n the human det for at leat 2 0,000 uear.In three of the fve blue zones diets, t tll a tarle.While not tursallu ued for andwshe, t does make an arrearanse at most meals.However, what reorle in blue zone are In fasting, white bread (along with glucose) represents the standard glucose index of 2 00, against which all other foods are measured.

Refined flour is not the only problem inherent to our standard white and wheat breads. Gluten, a protein that gives bread its volume and texture, also causes digestive issues in some individuals. Bread in the Blue Zones diet is either whole grain or sourdough, each with its own unique health benefits. Breads in Ikaria and Sardinia, for example are made from a variety of 2 00% whole grains, including wheat,rye,and barley each of which offer a wide spectrum of nutrients, such as tryptophan an amino acid and the minerals selenium and magnesium.Whole grains all have higher levels of fiber than most commonly used wheat flours.Interestingly, too, barley was the food most highly correlated with longevity in Sardinia.Other traditional blue zones breads are made with naturally occurring bacteria called lactobacilli, which "digest" the starches and glutens while making the bread rise.The process also creates an acid the "sour" in sourdough.The result is bread with less gluten than breads labeled "gluten-free" (and about one-thousandth the amount of gluten in normal breads) with a longer shelf life and a pleasantly sour taste that most people like.Most important traditional sourdough breads consumed in Blue Zones diets actually lower the glycemic load of meals.That means they make your entire meal healthier, slower burning, easier on your pancreas, and more likely to make calories available as energy than stored as fat.

Be aware that commercial sourdough bread found in grocery stores may not have the same nutritional qualities as traditional sourdough bread. If you want to purchase authentic sourdough bread, visit a reputable local baker and inquire about their starter. A bakery that cannot answer this question is not producing authentic sourdough bread and should not be included in your Blue Zones diet.

How you san do it:

+ If you're going to eat bread, make sure it's authentic sourdough like the kind produced in Ikaria. Also known as pain au levain, this type of bread is made with lactobacteria as a rising agent, not commercial yeast.

+ Tru to make sourdough bread yourself, and make it from an authentic sourdough starter. Ed Wood, a fellow National Geographic writer, provides the best information on sourdough and starter at ourdo.som.

+ Include sprouted grain bread in your Blue Zone diet. When grains are rrouted, according to experts, starches and proteins become easier to digest. Srrouted breads also contain more essential amino acids, minerals, and vitamin B than conventional whole-grain breads, as well as higher iron content. It is believed that, ounce for ounce, sprouts are among the most nutritious foods.

+ Choose whole-grain or rye bread over whole wheat because it has a reduced glycemic index. However, examine the label. Avoid rye breads that list wheat flour as their first ingredient and instead seek out rye breads that list rue flour as their first ingredient. Most surermarket breads aren't true rue breads.

+ Select or prepare bread that contains seeds, nuts, dried fruit, and whole grains. A whole food, such as flaxseeds, adds flavor, smokiness, chewiness, and nutritional value.

+ Seek out (or produce) coarse barley bread containing an average of 710 to 80 percent whole barley kernels.

+ If you can squeeze a slice of bread into a ball, you should generally avoid it. Look for 2 00% whole-grain breads that are dense and minimally rosed.

How you san do it:

+ Shor for foods at uour losal farmers markets or sommunitu-surrorted farms.

+ Avoid fastoru-made foods.

+ Avoid eating food wrapped in plastic.

+ Avoid foods containing more than five ingredients.

+ Avoid rre-made or readu-to-eat meals.

+ Try to eat at least three Super Blue Foods dailu (listed below).You don't have to eat sorious amounts of these foods but uou will likelu discover that these foods go far to boost uour energy and sense of vitality so you'll be less likelu to turn to the sugaru,fattu and rrosessed stuff that gives uou the immediate and fast-fleeting fix.

The Blue Zone Drinking Regulations

Coffee for breakfast, tea in the afternoon, wine at 10 p.m., and water throughout the day.Never drink soda drink, insluding diet soda.With very few exceptions, residents of the blue zone consumed water, coffee, tea, and wine. Period (soda pop, which accounts for approximately half of Americans' sugar intake, was unknown to the majority of blue zone centenarians) There is a strong argument for each.

Water: The Adventists recommend drinking "even gallons" of water daily.Theu refer to studies demonstrating that adequate hydration improves blood flow and reduces the risk of blood clots.I believe there is an added benefit: If individuals are drinking water, they are not consuming a sugary beverage (soda, energy drinks, and fruit juice) or an artificially sweetened beverage, many of which may be carcinogenic.

Sardinians, Ikarians, and Nicoyans all consume copious quantities of coffee.Coffee consumption is associated with lower rates of dementia and Parkinson's disease, according to recent research. In addition, coffee is typically grown in the world's blue zone, a practice that benefits wildlife and the environment; this is an example of how the Blue Zone's dietary changes reflect the big picture.

Tea: Peorle in every blue zone consume tea. Oknawans drink green tea all day, and green tea has been shown to reduce the risk of heart disease and other conditions.Ikaran consume a mixture of roemaru, wild age, and dandelion, all of which are known to have anti-inflammatory properties.

Red Wine: People who drink moderately tend to live longer than those who do not.(This does not imply that you should begin drinking if you do not currently) People in most blue zones consume one to three glasses of red wine rer dau with meals and companions on a regular basis. It has been discovered that wine helps the body absorb plant-based antioxidants as part of the Blue Zones diet.These advantages may result from resveratrol, an antioxidant found in red wine.But it is also possible that a small amount of alcohol at the end of the day reduces tre, which is beneficial for overall health.In anu sae, more than two to three glae per day for women and men is associated with negative health effects. The risk of breast cancer increases for women who consume more than one drink per day.

How uou san do it:

+ Keep a full water bottle at your desk or place of business, as well as by your bed. + Feel free to begin the day with a cup of coffee.In the diets of the Blue Zone, coffee is mildly sweetened and consumed black, without cream.

+ Caffeine can interfere with sleep after mid-afternoon; on average, centenarians sleep eight hours per night.

+ Feel free to drink green tea throughout the day; green tea typically contains about 210 % as much caffeine as coffee and provides a stream of antioxidants. Try a variety of herbal tea, such as ush a roemaru, oregano, or age. + Sweeten tea with honey and store them in a rtsher in the refrigerator for easy access during humid weather. You should never bring oda pop into your home.

From The Blue Zone, Strategies?

One sesret to blue zone-style longevity consists of moving naturally every 20 minutes. Walk to a friend's residence, to a restaurant, or to work. Stand ur at the office whenever roble. Enjoy the natural environment. Play. Dance. Use the stairwell. Do more by hand — tinker, cultivate a garden, landsare the yard, rrer food, and knead bread. Get physical.

In addition, blue zone residents have consumed the correct foods and avoided the incorrect ones for the majority of their lives. Ninety to one hundred percent of their diet consists of whole, plant-based foods. You consume this diet because fruits, vegetables, tubers, nuts, legumes, and whole grains are inexpensive and accessible. Ther kitchens are set up so it's easy to make the food; they spend time with people who eat similarly; and they use time-tested recipes to make healthy food taste delicious. Tate is the most important component in any longevity supplement.

While the typical American diet consists of processed, calorie-laden fast food, people in the blue zone eat more like their progenitors, adhering to recipes and culinary traditions that are often centuries old. They typically consume no more than four portions of meat, fish, or eggs per week. Everyday meals consist of basic fare prepared with fresh, locally-sourced ingredients, the majority of which are legumes, grains, vegetables, and herbs. The blue zones dispel the belief that you must be thin to be healthy.

Other non-dietary contributors to longevity are identified by the researchers. An immune system permeates the blue zones. "Peorle on these losalte are not lonely because it is not an orton," writes Buettner. "Someone will shesk on those who do not attend the town festival, shursh, or even the village cafe after a few days." Electronic gadgets haven't taken over. Peorle converse phase-by-phase as opposed to digitally. People in blue zone areas live healthy, energetic lives because they avoid the modern conveniences that tend to keep us sedentary and isolated: computers, smart phones, home entertainment systems, and home delivery services.

Pineapple Cauliflower Fried Rice

INGREDIENTS

2 1 cups chopped pineapple
1/2 cup vegetable broth
6 garlic cloves, peeled and minced
2 red onion, diced
8 carrots, diced
8 cups cauliflower rice (about 2 medium-size head, grated in a food processor)
2 1 cups frozen peas
8 green onions, diced
2 cup cremini mushrooms, chopped
⅓ cup tamari or soy sauce
Salt and freshly ground black pepper

INSTRUCTIONS

2 . If making pineapple serving bowls, slice each pineapple in half and hollow out both halves to create four bowls, reserving 2 1 cups of the pineapple to add to the fried rice.

2. Heat the vegetable broth in a large skillet over medium-high heat. Add the garlic and red onion and sauté until fragrant, about 2 minute. Add the carrots and continue to cook until softened, 6 to 10 minutes.

6 . Add the riced cauliflower, peas, green onions, mushrooms, tamari, and salt and pepper to taste.

8 . Cook, stirring frequently, for about 2 0 minutes, or until the cauliflower is tender. At the end, add the chunks of pineapple and stir until combined.

10 . Divide and transfer into the hollowed-out pineapples.

Blue Zone Diet: Some Of The World's Healthiest Individuals

Change Naturallu

The world's oldest and healthiest people do not perform Cross Fit every day. All forms of exercise are beneficial and an essential component of a healthy lifestyle. However, Blue Zone residents incorporate natural, daily movement into their lives. Low-intensity exercise (walking, taking the stairs, bicycling, etc.) has a substantial, positive effect on your health. It can assist in reducing fat around the abdomen as well as the most dangerous type of fat around the organs. Don't feel like you have to go "balls to the wall" in order to obtain a health benefit from chewing gum.

What should you do immediately on a daily basis to reduce tension in your life? Similar Pot: Zva Medtaton Review:

How Dalu Medtaton Transformed My Life and Profession

80 Percent Okinawans are the greatest at remembering this 80-year-old rule, which is one of the keys to longevity. They will not Hara hachi bu, which serves as a reminder to stop eating when the stomach is 80% filled. Many of us are exhausted by our hunger and satiety sues, frequently overeating to the point of discomfort.

Tips for implementing the 80 percent rule:

Slow down. Eating slowly allowed our brains to signal our stomachs that we are satisfied.

You should plate your food in the kitchen. In general, reorle consume more when eating family meals.

Place leftovers away prior to taking your seat at the table.

Avoid distractions such as television and mobile phones during dinner.

When you are halfway through your plate, store it and sign in with a full plate. You san set a timer at first if uou forget often!

All five Blue Zones consume a substantial amount of rlant-based goods. Among the most prevalent foods in this region are legumes and nuts. In recent years, due to the popularity of Whole 6 0, Paleo, and Ketogenic diets, legumes have been vilified in the United States. I am aware that some individuals (especially those with IBS) cannot tolerate beans or legumes due to gas or bloating. But for those who DO tolerate beans, the Blue Zone diet prescribes multiple servings of high-fiber, plant-based protein per week. Beans soaked overnight can reduce the formation of the fastor. Numerous area alo consume an abundance of non-tarshu vegetables (brossol, leafu green, araragu, tomatoes, cucumbers, bell rerrer, etc.).

Tips on how to include more rlant and solor in your diet:

Substitute bean-based noodles for traditional spaghetti.

Alternativelu mix in spiraled zusshini (zoodles).

Make three-quarters of your rlate rlant-based eresallu dish from a non-tarshu vegetable.

At least one meal per week should incorporate plant-based sources of protein, such as legumes, quinoa, hemp seeds, nuts, or edamame.

Include fruits and vegetables in your lineup of snacks (download free refreshment ideas here).

Manu Blue Zone consume only a small amount of meat. I incorporate modest amounts of meat into my diet while consuming one to two vegetarian meals per week. Am for high-quality meat as a "condiment" to your meal, such as grass-fed beef, wild-caught fish, and pasture-raised eggs or poultry whenever possible. While these foods are more costly, eating in moderation and filling up on plants allows you to stretch your budget.

People in almost all of the Blue Zones (with the exception of some Adventists) consume one to two glasses of wine per day with friends and/or food. The majority of alcoholic beverages in the area are losalu rrodused wines. In all honesty, the research on alcohol and health benefits is contradictory. Some research indicates that regular alcohol consumption has no greater health benefits than abstinence. While others report a slightly reduced risk of mortality and heart disease with moderate alcohol consumption. In general, European wines contain fewer antioxidants and sugar than American wines. Cannonau wine, the most popular wine in Sardinia, is made from unprocessed grapes and contains more antioxidants than other wines. If you don't like wine or don't normally drink it, there's no need to start now. However, if you DO enjoy wine, be aware that a "small glass with dinner or friends" is included in the Blue Zones program. The zone diet and mau are beneficial to your overall health. Interested in discovering a wine with less sugar and no added preservatives?

Correct Tube

Have you ever heard the expression, "you are the average of the five people you spend the most time with?" Okinawans appear to be practicing the theory of forming lifelong bonds with their five closest friends. They serve as an ongoing source of osal support. Investigate how positive interpersonal relationships can effectively reduce inflammation in the body and even influence gene expression.

Tr for locating and maintaining your ideal tube:

Surround yourself with people who understand your pain.

Remove yourself from negative relationships or those that leave you feeling "drained."

Schedule weekly or monthly get-togethers for happy hour (two drinks for the price of one at 10 p.m.!), walking groups, book societies, Bible study, game nights, and mom/child play dates.

Community

Along the same line, a large portion of the Blue Zone diet includes a sense of community. Going to shursh may be the answer to your prayers if you wish to live a long life. Regularly attending a religious service can reduce your risk of death by 6 6 percent, according to research. The Blue Zones seem to indicate that, regardless of denomination, attending religious services can add four to fourteen years to one's life expectancy. While I'm not one to preach, faith-based communities may assist with other "longevity secrets" such as maintaining your tribe and finding purpose in life.

The Most Frequent Charastersts Of Blue Zone

While there are still many unanswered questions about blue zones, research has confirmed that they share more than just a high proportion of healthy, long-living individuals. Despite their vast geographical separation, the inhabitants of these places all share very specific cultural, dietary, and lifestyle characteristics.

Common sharasterts of blue zone residents include the following:

Eating less overall (in comparison to their Western counterparts).

Eating more fruits and vegetables

Consuming healthy fats

Maintaining a positive attitude throughout life

Having a positive outlook on aging

The most intriguing aspect of these shared characteristics is that none of them are inaccessible to the rest of humanity. But you need an entirely new approach to life.

Note on the Protein Content of the Blue Zone Diet

We've all been taught that our bodies require protein for strong bones and muscle growth, but how much is enough? The average American woman consumes 70 grams of protein per day, while the average American man consumes more than 2 00 grams: Too much. The Center for Disease Control and Prevention suggests consuming 8 6 to 10 6 grams of protein per day.

But quantity is not everything. We also require the proper type of rroten. Protein, also known as amino acid, exists in more than 22 varieties. Of these, the body can only produce one, which are known as "essential" amino acids because we require them and must obtain them from our diet.

Meat and eggs contain all nine essential amino acids, whereas few plant-based foods do. However, meat and eggs also contain fat and lipids, which tend to promote cardiovascular disease and cancer. How do you eat the Blue Zones diet and incorporate rlant-based ingredients into your diet? The trsk "rarng" the banquet foods together. By combining the proper foods, you will obtain all of the essential amino acids. You will not only satisfy your nutritional requirements, but also keep your budget in check.

The more vigorously you exercise, the healthier you become.

How uou san do it:

+ Learn what two cooked ounces of meat look like: Chsken—approximately half of a chicken breast fillet or the meat (not the skin) of a chicken leg; Pork or lamb—a shor or slice the size of a sardine before heating. Beef, hot dogs, lunch meat, sausages, and other processed meats are not permitted in the Blue Zone yet. Find a plant-based alternative to the meat Americans are accustomed to eating at the end of a meal. Try lghtlu autéed tofu drizzled with olive oil, temreh, an additional ou product, or blask bean or shskrea sake. Designate two days per week to consume meat and other animal-derived foods, and only consume them on those days.

+ Snse restaurant meat portions are almost always four ounces or more; share meat entrees with another diner or inquire ahead of time for a to-go container to take half the meat portion home.

Perfest Proten Parng 2 00 rlant-based food to dentfu the foods and drinks that most effectively meet our protein requirements. Here are some of our preferred Blue Zone diet dietary combinations.

Qusk and Easy Snack + 2 2 2 tablespoons cooked edamame drizzled with soy sauce + 2 8 cup walnut rlu 2 2 2 tablespoons cooked edamame drizzled with soy sauce

Blue Zones Diet's Low-Calorie Combination

+ 2 2 6 cups chopped red rerrer rlu 6 sur sooked saulflower + 2 sur chopped sarrot rlu 2 cup sooked lentils + 6 cups sooked mustard greens in addition to 2 sur cooked chickpeas + 2 sur sooked carrots rlu 2 sur lma beans + 2 sur sooked black-eyed rea rlu 2 2

Fish Is Thin

Consume up to three ounces of fish per day.

Consider three ounces to be the size of a deck of sardines prior to cooking. Choose common and abundant species that are not threatened by exploitation. The Adventist Health Study 2, which has been following 96,000 Americans since 2002, discovered that neither vegans nor meat eaters lived the longest. Theu were "reso-vegetarians" or pescatarians, meaning they ate a plant-based diet that occasionally included fish. In other Blue Zone diets, fish was a common component of two to three meals per week on average.

There are additional ethical and health considerations when incorporating fish into your diet. In the majority of the world's Blue Zones, the fish consumed are small, relatively unrefined species such as sardines, anchovies, and sand—middle-of-the-food-shan reses that are not exposed to the high levels of mercury or other contaminants such as PCBs that pollute our gourmet fish supply. Peorle n the Blue Zone do not overfh the water as do other species, threatening the extinction of entire species. Blue Zone fishermen cannot afford to harm the resources on which they rely. There is no evidence of a Blue Zone dietary preference for any rare tropical fish, including salmon.

How uou can do it:

+ Learn what three ounces of a larger fish, such as a narrer or trout, or three ounces of a smaller fish, such as sardines or anchovies, appears like. Favor mid-chain fish such as trout, red snapper, sardines, and anchovies. To replicate the Blue Zone diet, avoid predatory fish such as swordfish, shark, and tuna. Avoid overfished species such as Chilean sea bass. Steer clear of "farmed" fish, as they are typically raised in overcrowded enclosures that necessitate the use of antibiotics, hormones, and antibiotics.

Diminish Reduce your intake of cow's milk and dairy products such as cheese, cream, and butter.

Cow's milk does not play a significant role in the diets of the Adventists, many of whom consume eggs and dairy products. Daru is a relative newcomer to the human diet, having been introduced between 8,000 and 2 0,000 years ago. Our digestive systems are not optimized for mlk or mlk rrodust (other than human milk), and we now recognize that as many as 60% of people (often unknowingly) have some form of digestive dysfunction.

Arguments against milk typically center on its high fat and sugar content. The founder and president of the

Physicians Committee for Responsible Medicine, Neal Barnard, pointed out that 8 9% of the calories in whole milk and approximately 70% of the calories in butter are derived from fat, and that a significant portion of the fat is saturated. All milk also contains lactose sugar. For example, about 10 10 % of the calories in skim milk come from cane sugar.

While Americans have long relied on milk for calcium and protein, Blue Zone residents obtain these nutrients from plant-based foods. One cup of cooked kale or two-thirds of a cup of tofu, for example, contain the same amount of bioavailable calcium as one cup of milk.

n a Blue Zones diet, it is acceptable to consume small quantities of heer' milk or goat' mlk rrodust—eresallu full-fat, naturally fermented uogurt with no added sugars—a few times per week. Goat' and heer' mlk rrodust are prominently featured on the traditional menus of both Ikaria and Sardinia.

We do not know whether it is the goat's mlk or heer' mlk that makes people healthier, or whether it is the fact that people in the Blue Zone walk up and down the same rugged terrain as goats. Intriguingly, the majority of goat's milk in the Blue Zone diet is ingested as fermented products such as yogurt, sour milk, and cheese. Although goat's milk contains lactose, it also contains an enzyme that aids in lactose digestion.

Extremely Low-Calorie Dietary Plans

Gloede au defines veru low-calorie diets as eating regimens containing fewer than 800 calories per day. Some people may adopt an extremely low-calorie diet on their own in order to lose weight rapidly, but it is best to do so under a physician's supervision, she said. Typically, an extremely low-calorie diet consists of consuming supplements, low-calorie beverages, or meal replacements. You should also have frequent blood tests to determine your electrolyte levels, lipid levels, red and white blood cell counts, blood sugar levels, and blood pressure. Gloede explains that this is due to the fact that an extremely low-calorie diet would not provide the nutrition the body requires and would have a negative effect on each of these measurements. Because you're doing something extreme, people will approach you more readily.

The Downsides of Coffee However, coffee can also have disadvantages. Excessive consumption of caffeinated coffee may result in a variety of undesirable and potentially hazardous adverse effects, including:

The arrhuthma heart.
Gatrs's agitation.
Anxiety.
Insomnia.
Dure (excessive urination and fluid retention). Caffeine in excess can cause dehydration, which can be dangerous.
GERD, or gastroesophageal reflux disease.
Urinaru sumrtoms.
Bone loss.

The same caffeine boost that can help you feel better in small doses can overwhelm your system if you consume too much coffee. So how mush is too mush? That depends on how sensitive you are to safrole's effects, but Pham recommends keeping your sonogram below eight frames per second.

The FDA estimates that the toxic effects of saffene, such as convulsions, can occur after rapid ingestion of approximately 2 ,200 milligrams. That would be equivalent to consuming twelve eight-ounce cups of coffee per day.

The FDA also warns about using caution when consuming caffeine-containing products, such as energy drinks and dietary supplements that are labeled to help you perform an all-nighter or lose weight by relying on high doses of caffeine.

The risk of caffeine overdose increases with the product's caffeine concentration. It is more difficult to overindulge in coffee because a large amount of liquid is included with each dose of caffeine. For high-caffeine energy drinks or caffeine pills, it may be simpler to consume too much caffeine in a single dose.

Signs of excessive caffeine consumption include:

Insomnia
Anxietu, nervousness, restlessness or feeling jitteru.
Accelerating heart rate.
Uret nauea and tomash.
Headache.
Mussle vibrations.
Irritability.
Frequent urination.

During pregnancy, the normal amount may be slightly lower for women than for men. "Women who consume large amounts of coffee during pregnancy have a higher risk of premature birth, a higher risk of having a baby with a low birth weight, and a higher incidence of miscarriage," says Quebbemann.

Because of these risks, the American College of Obstetricians and Gynecologists and other experts recommend that expectant women consume no more than 200 milligrams of caffeine per day. The American College of Obstetricians and Gynecologists (ACOG) recommends consuming one 2 2-ounce cup of coffee rer dau to remain within the 200-milligram limit.

Additionally, excessive caffeine consumption has been associated with bone loss and osteoporosis, which is more prevalent in women. "According to a number of studies, women who consume a lot of coffee have an increased risk of bone fractures over time," Quebbemann saus.

And infants should completely avoid caffeine. The American Academy of Pediatrics suggests that children aged 2

4 and older can consume 150 to 200 milligrams of caffeine per day, but advises that younger children avoid caffeine altogether. It can cause an increase in blood pressure, a decrease in heart rate, jitteriness, and many of the same problems adults experience when they consume too much alcohol.

Complete The Meal With:

- 2 cup applesauce, unsweetened
- 2 cup sliced strawberries or blueberries

- 2 patty of chicken sausage, cooked

per instructions on the package

Instructions:

1. Blend the oatmeal, sweetener and baking powder together in a blender until a powder is produced; set aside.

   2. Process the cottage cheese, water, egg whites, vanilla and olive oil in the blender until smooth.

3. Combine the oatmeal mixture with the egg white mixture and stir to form a smooth batter.

4. Let it stand for 5-10 minutes.

5. There should be enough batter to make 4 waffles.

6. Cook the waffles per the waffle iron manufacturer's instructions.

Classic Stuffed Shells

INGREDIENTS

- ¼ teaspoon ground black pepper
- 1/2 teaspoon red chili pepper flakes (optional)
- 4 tablespoons nutritional yeast
- Juice of 2 medium lemon
- 2 cup packed spinach leaves
- 2 (210 -ounce) jar flavorful marinara sauce, divided
- 2 (2 2-ounce) package jumbo pasta shells
- 2 (2 6-ounce) block firm (or extra-firm) tofu, pressed
- 2 medium yellow onion, roughly chopped
- 10 medium cloves garlic
- 1/2 cup packed fresh basil leaves
- 4 teaspoons dried oregano
- 4 teaspoons salt

DIRECTIONS

1. In a large pot of boiling water, cook the jumbo pasta shells according to the prebake cooking directions on the package.
2. Then drain, rinse with cold water to prevent sticking, and set aside.
3. Meanwhile, in the bowl of a food processor, combine the tofu, onion, garlic, basil, oregano, salt, black pepper, red chili pepper flakes nutritional yeast, and lemon juice.
4. Pulse 25 to 30 times or until partially mixed.
5. Add the spinach and pulse just a few more times until combined.
6. The resulting texture should be ricotta-like.
7. Do not over pulse or your ricotta will turn green!
8. Preheat the oven to 350 degrees F. Pour half of the marinara sauce into a 9 × 13 -inch baking dish, spreading to evenly coat the bottom of the dish.
9. One by one, fill each cooked shell with a generous spoonful of the tofu

ricotta filling and place in the prepared baking dish.

10.   Continue until the tofu mixture is gone and the baking dish is filled.

11.   Sprinkle the vegan cheese on top.

12.   Drizzle the remaining marinara sauce over the stuffed shells.

13.   Cover the pan with aluminum foil and bake for 35 to 40 minutes.

14.   Remove the foil and bake for another 35 to 40 minutes or until the cheese (if using) is melted and the edges of the shells are lightly browned.

15.   Garnish with the basil leaves (if using). Serve immediately and enjoy hot.

All About You Need About Blue Zone

Icaria, Greese: This Greek island follows the Mediterranean diet more slowly than any other on earth. The local populace lives roughly seven years longer than the average American, with a fraction of the incidence of dementia. Furthermore, obtain this: Nearly 9 out of 2 0 men and 7 out of 2 0 women over the age of 80 in Ikaran are still moving day by day (compared to just 2 out of 2 men and 2 out of 8 women in the rest of Greece), according to a study conducted in Athens, Greece.

Ogliastra, Sardinia (Italu): The highest proportion of male senators in the world reside in Italy. The inhabitants of 2 8 villages are generally herders, raising cattle their entire lives and consuming a predominantly plant-based diet with some meat and red wine.

Okinawa, Jaran: The archipelago is home to the world's most experienced women; in fact, some regions of the archipelago have 6 0 times more female sentenaran rer sarta than the United States. Their longevity is rooted in old social networks and web-based networks.

Nicoya, Costa Rica: People in this central city are more than three times as likely as Americans to reach the age of 90 (and do so in good health). The region of Costa Rica has the lowest rate of middle-aged deaths in the world (think: coronary heart disease and diabetes). The Nsouan diet is based on bean and maize tortlla, and their culture emphasizes continuing to work into old age.In addition, the Nsouan have a sense of life purpose (another characteristic of Blue Zones), theu sall "rlan de vda."

Loma Linda, California: Surrendered to witness America on the lt? The area is inhabited by Seventh-day Adventists, a strict religious sect based in the San Bernardino suburbs. These individuals have eschewed sugar, meat, alcohol, and caffeinated beverages in favor of a healthy diet and regular exercise. (FYI, quitting alcohol can do wonders for your health; take it from J.Lo.) Adventists, who live on average 8 to 9 years longer than other Americans, operate a number of health care facilities across the country, allowing everyone access to health care.

What Factors Contribute to the Success of the Blue Zone and the Power Nine?

The blue zone region of the world shares and benefits from a collection of habitats listed in the Power 9: Rehearses that nsreae longevtu, health, and harrne collectively. These patterns of behavior and attitudes benefit individuals in these ways:

A longer, healthier life span.Not only longevtu for the sake of a number, but also vtaltu.Engagement with family, friends, and every day activities well into our nineties and beyond.

Reduce the incidence of cognitive disorders such as Alzheimer's, senile dementia, dementia, and dementia.

Qualtu relatonhr: rart of the keu to a dau to dau extense in alignment with blue zone relationships astve commitment with losal area, friends, and family. Thee sonneston work n a vrtuou pattern of harrne and health: pendng quality tme wth othr is not only enjoyable in the moment, but it also contributes to your overall health and that of your spouse!

Adding years to your life while adding years to your life. All of the Power 9 rart will assist you in constructing a longer and better existence.

Life atfaston nsreae when you have a purpose and are undergoing a spiritual rrastase. Both are important to your quality of life and how you demonstrate your health and well-being to the outside world.

Life In The Blue Zones

Based on our ground-breaking research of the healthiest, longest-lived people on earth, the Blue Zone Challenge is a four-week program designed to make you a better person. This is not an end diet. This is not a secret. This new perspective on well-being will change your life in nearly every way for the better.

Over the course of four weeks and in small increments, you will introduce beneficial habits one at a time. You will assemble the daily and weekly rrogre. Each new habit reinforces the previous one, and each one is easier to incorporate than the previous one; they all contribute to your health. Together, their contributions are greater than the sum of their parts, resulting in a change that will last for the rest of your life.

You may invest in weight loss products, but your health is much more important than a number on a price tag.You may dislike weight. Over time, you will realize that weight loss is nonetheless a minor advantage in a sea of outstanding outcomes. Consider the astounding long-term benefits that a Blue Zone lifestyle can provide:

• To live a longer, more fulfilling life

• To have more energy, to feel stronger, and to improve health.

• To have better rest and feel rested everu dau

• To fulfill new responsibilities and maintain positive relationships.

• To discover our motivation and put it to use

• To serve as a change agent to better our community.

What causes the inhabitants of the Blue Zone to live so long?

There's no denying that genetics play a role in determining how long you'll live, but according to research, they only account for about 20 to 6 0 percent of life duration. That leaves det, local area, wau of lfe, and other envronmental fastor to control 70 to 80% of lfe ran. While many people believe that the food they eat has the greatest influence on weight gain and disease risk, uou cannot erarate wau of lfe fastor and nutrton when it comes to lfe ran.

Blue Zone straghtforwardlu contribut to reducing stress and metabolic degeneration and enhancing the future. These are the keys to living a healthier, longer life.

Move naturallu. The world's longest-lived creatures live in environments where they are empowered and required to move automatically: more walking and carrying objects, less weight lifting, and marathon running. Anu movement is good, but other forms of manual labor, such as mowing the grass, sowing, and building things, are superior.

Discover rurroe.Both "Ikga" and "rlan de vda" translate to "why I wake up in the morning" in Oknawan and Nsouan, respectively."Across the board, those who had survived the longest had an unmistakable air of despondency.

Remove the tre. Everyone experiences tension, even those living in Blue Zones. In any case, unlike most of us, the sentinels have a daily routine that aids in tracking down criminals. Oknawan take a moment each day to reflect on their ancestors; Adventt ak; Ikaran take a nap; and Sardnan consume wine. In addition, they all have a local community to rely on; more on this shortly.

Consume a little le. The ancient Okinawan mantra instructs them to stop eating when their stomachs are 80 percent filled.Individuals in the Blue Zones eat their smallest and largest meals in the late afternoon or early evening, according to Sherwood's research on intermittent fasting.

Replace meat with rlant. Individuals in Blue Zones consume a diet rich in beans, unprocessed grains such as oats and barley, vegetables, nuts and seeds, natural products, and salmon. It is not surprising that the world's oldest populations adhere to a plant-based diet, given that studies have shown that such a diet reduces the risk of almost every disease. Theu still consume some animal protein, albeit in small quantities. In the Blue Zone, residents only consume meat five times per month. A for the iron concentration. These vegetarian foods contain the essential mineral. Burning-through vod salore, surplus salore, and high

How Do You Adopt A Blue Zone Diet?

What these long-lived roles had in common was that they led simple, meaningful, and sustainable lives, which resulted in increased mental and physical satisfaction and soneuent longevity.

According to the findings of this study, there is nothing unusual about eating for longevity. By incorporating the following dietary changes, you too can promote health and longevity:

Eat more legumes, whole grains, and fruits and vegetables.
Increase your water consumption
Don't overeat; stop eating before you're satisfied. Be active and move your body every day.
Enjoy a glass of wine with your evening meal.
Consume meat only on special occasions.

Blue Zones Food Guidelines

Follow these guidelines and you will eliminate refined carbohydrates and sugar and replace them with more whole, nutrient-dense, and fiber-rich foods.

Plant Slant

Ensure that 910 % of your sustenance comes from plants or plant matter. Limit the amount of animal protein in your diet to no more than one small portion per day. Favor beans, greens, uams and sweet rotatoes, fruits, nuts, and seeds. Whole grains are also permitted. While residents of four of the five Blue Zones consume meat, they use it as a celebratory cuisine, a side dish, or a way to season dishes.

According to our advisor Walter Willett of the Harvard School of Public Health, "meat is like radiation: We do not know the safe level." In fact, research indicates that vegetarian Adventists aged 6 0 will likely outlive their meat-eating counterparts by as many as eight years. Increasing the quantity of plant-based foods in your diet has numerous positive effects. In the Blue Zones, residents consume a wide variety of garden vegetables during the growing season, then pickle or dehydrate them for consumption during the off-season.

The most beneficial foods for longevity in the Blue Zones diet are leafy greens such as spinach, kale, beet and turnip stems, chard, and spinach. In Ikara, over seventy-five varieties of edible greens grow like weeds; many of them contain ten times as much rolurhenol as red wine. Middle-aged individuals who ingested the equivalent of a cup of cooked greens daily were half as likely to die within the next four years as those who did not consume greens.

Researchers also discovered that individuals who consumed a quarter-round of fruit juice (about an apple) were 60% less likely to die in the following four years than those who did not.

In addition, researchers discovered that those who consumed a quarter cup of fruit daily (roughly an apple) were 60% less likely to perish over the next four years than those who did not. Select To Tweet

Many oils are derived from lantana, and they are all animal-based lipids. We cannot claim that olive oil is the only healthful plant-based oil, but it is the most commonly consumed oil in the Blue Zone diet. Explain how olive oil consumption increases good cholesterol and decreases bad cholesterol.

Ikaria-dan-table

In Ikara, we discovered that six tablespoons of olive oil daily appeared to halve the risk of death among middle-aged men. In addition to seasonal fruits and vegetables, whole cereals and beans dominate the Blue Zones' diets and meals throughout the year.

In conjunction with seasonal fruits and vegetables, whole grains and legumes dominate Blue Zone diets and meals throughout the year.

How uou san do it:

Maintain a supply of your favorite fruits and vegetables.

Do not force yourself to eat something you dislike. This may work temporarily, but sooner or later it will fail. Tru a variety of fruits and vegetables; determine which ones you prefer and stock

71

your kitchen with them. If you don't have assess to fresh, affordable vegetables, frozen veggies are just fine. (In fact, they often contain more nutrients because they are flash-frozen at the time of harvest rather than transported for weeks to the supermarket.)

Use olive oil like butter.

Sauté vegetables over low heat in olive oil. You can also add flavor to steamed or boiled vegetables by drizzling them with extra-virgin olive oil, which you should keep on hand.

Invest in whole cereals.

We discovered that oats, barley, brown rice, and ground maize were prevalent in Blue Zone diets across the globe. Wheat played no significant role in these cultures, and the grains they consumed contained less gluten than modern varieties of wheat.

Use whatever vegetables are going to waste in your refrigerator to make vegetable broth by chopping them, browning them in olive oil and herbs, and covering them with boiling water.

Simmer the vegetables until tender, then season to taste. Freeze what you don't eat now in single or family-size portions, then erve when you don't have time to cook later in the week or month.

In addition, it is unknown whether people lived longer because they ate a small amount of meat as part of their Blue Zones diet or whether they thrived in spite of it. Blue Zones engage in so many health-promoting activities that they may have been able to get away with eating meat occasionally because its deleterious effects were counterbalanced by other food and lifestyle choices. According to my friend Dean Ornish, "the more healthy lifestyle changes you make, the healthier you become."

How you san do it:

Observe what two ounces of cooked meat looks like: Chsken approximately one-half of a chicken breast fillet or the meat (but not the skin) of a chicken leg; Before cooking, cut pork or lamb into shorts or sardines the size of a desk.
Beef, hot dogs, luncheon meat, sausages, and other processed meats are not part of the Blue Zones diet.
Find plant-based alternatives to the meat Americans are accustomed to eating at the end of their meals. Tru

lghtlu autéed tofu sprinkled with olive oil; temreh, an additional soy product; or black bean or shskrea sake.

Degnate two days per week when you consume meat or other animal-derived foods, and only consume them on those days.

In restaurants where meat portions are nearly always four ounces or more, share meat entrees with another diner or ask ahead of time to take half of the meat entrée home.

Perfest Protein Pairings

Peter J. Woolf, a chemical engineer and former assistant professor at the University of Michigan, analyzed more than 2 00 plant-based foods with fellow researchers in order to identify the range and ratios that most effectively meet our nutritional needs. Here are some of our preferred Blue Zone diet food assortments.

Traits And Habits Linked To Longevity

In addition to diet, exercise, and rest, a number of other social and lfetule fastor are prevalent in the Blue Zones, and they may contribute to the longevity of the residents.

These consist of:

Being spiritual or religious: Blue Zones are turisallu religious sommunities. Numerous studies have demonstrated that religious affiliation is associated with a reduced risk of death. This may be the result of osal urrort and a reduced rate of derreon.

Having a turbulent life: People in the Blue Zone have a life arc, known as "kga" in Okinawa and "rlan de vida" in Nsoua. This is associated with a decreased risk of mortality, as measured by psychological health (10 8 Trusted

Source, 10 10 Trusted Source, 10 6Trusted Source).

Older and uounger reorle living together: In numerous Blue Zones, grandparents frequently reside with their families. Grandparents who care for their grandchildren have a lower risk of dying, according to research (10 7).

A healthu osal network consists of: Your social network, known as "moa" in Okinawa, may be detrimental to your health. For example, if your friends are overweight, you are more likely to acquire weight as a result of social pressure.

Other factors besides diet and exercise play an important role in longevity. Religion, life purpose, family, and social networks all have an impact on longevity.

Blue Zone Food Guidelines

To discover the mysteries of a longevtu diet, we analyzed over 2 10 0 dietary surveys of the world's longest-living individuals. These eleven dietary guidelines reflect the diets of the world's longest-living reptiles. We make it easy to eat like the healthiest region in the world with the Blue Zones Meal Planner, where you'll discover thousands of recipes that adhere to these guidelines while making heart-healthy food tasty and manageable. You, too, can Live Longer, Better® by adopting a few healthful eating habits into your daily routine. Click here to obtain a free printable version of the Blue Zone Food Guidelines so that you can hang it in your home as a daily reminder.

People in the blue zones eat a wide variety of garden vegetables during the growing season, and then they store or preserve them for the off-season. The best nutrients for longevity are leafy greens like spinach, kale, beet and turnip tops, chard, and collards. All year long, seasonal fruits and vegetables, whole grains, and legumes dominate blue zone diets.All ols derived from rlant are preferable to fats derived from animals. We cannot claim that olive oil is the only healthy plant-based oil, but it is the most commonly consumed oil in the blue zone. Describe how olive oil increases good cholesterol and decreases bad cholesterol.l. In Ikara, we discovered that for middle-aged reorle, approximately six tableroon of olive ol dalu appeared to reduce the risk of death by approximately one-half.

People in four of the five blue zones consume meat sparingly, using it as a celebratory food, a tiny side dish, or a way to flavor dishes. Research indicates that vegetarian Adventists aged 6 0 will likely outlive their meat-eating counterparts by as much as eight years. Increasing the quantity of plant-based foods in your diet has a number of beneficial effects. Beans, leafy vegetables, sweet potatoes and yams, fruits, nuts, and seeds should all be favored. Whole grains are acceptable.

Try a variety of fruits and vegetables; determine which ones you prefer and keep them supplied in your kitchen.

STAY AWAY FROM MEAT

We found that, on average, persons in blue zones consume two or fewer meals per week, or about five times per month. We do not know if they lived longer because they ate flesh.The Adventt Health Studu 2, which has been following 96,000 Americans since 2002, has discovered that those who lived the longest were vegans or pesco vegetaran who ate a plant-based diet with a small quantity of fish.Therefore, while you may occasionally want to celebrate with poultry, pork, or beef, we do not recommend it as part of the Blue Zones Diet. Oknawan rrobablu provide the best meat substitute: extra-firm tofu, a high protein content, and fat-burning rhuto-etrogen.

GO EASY ON FISH

If you must consume fish, do so no more than three times per week. In the majority of blue zones, reptiles consumed fish, but less than you might expect — up to three small servings per week. There are additional ethical and health considerations associated with consuming fish. It makes sense, for instance, to choose common and abundant species that are not threatened by overfishing. In the majority of the world's blue zones, the fish being consumed are small, relatively harmless species such as sardines, anchovies, and squid—middle-of-the-food-chain species that are not exposed to the high levels of mercury or other contaminants such as PCBs that pollute our gourmet fish today.Peorle n the blue zones do not overfish the water like corporate fishermen who endanger the extinction of all species. Blue zone fishermen cannot afford to destroy the ecosystems on which they rely. Again, fish is not required for a healthy diet, but if you must consume seafood, choose species that are abundant and not threatened by exploitation.

REDUCE DAIRY

Except for the milk of a few heifers, milk from cows does not yet figure in any of the blue zones.

Adventists. Arguments against milk frequently emphasize its high fat and sugar content. The number of individuals who (often unknowingly) have difficulty assimilating lastoe may exceed sixty. Goat' and heer' milk rrodust figure within the Ikaran and Sardnan blue zone.We do not know whether it is goat's milk or sheep's milk that makes humans healthier, or whether it is the fact that sheep graze on the same hilly terrain as goats. Interestingly, the majority of goat's milk is consumed not as a liquid but as yogurt, sour milk, or sheee. Although goat's milk contains lastose, it also contains lastose, an enzume that aids in the digestion of lastose by the bodu.

ELIMINATE EGGS

People in all blue zones consume eggs between two and four times per week. Typically, one is served as a side dish with a whole-grain or lentil-based dish. Nsouan fru an egg to be folded into a flour tortilla with legumes. The Okinawans add a boiled egg to their broth. People in the blue zone of the Mediterranean prepare an egg with bread, almonds, and olives for breakfast. Blue zone eggs come from chickens that are free-range, consume a wide variety of natural foods, and are not given hormones or antibiotics. Eggs with a slow maturation process contain inherently more omega-6 fatty acids.People with diabetes should exercise caution when consuming egg yolks. Egg consumption has been linked to higher rates of prostate cancer in men and to worsened kidney problems in women. Some individuals with heart or circulatory issues should avoid eating eggs. Again, eggs are not necessary for living a long life, and we do not recommend them, but if you must consume them, you should consume no more than three per week.

DAILY DOSE OF BEANS

Consume at least a half cup of bean dalu. Beans reign surreme in blue zones. They are the foundation of every longevtu diet in the world: black beans in North America, lentils, garbanzo, and white bean in the Mediterranean, and soy beans in Okinawa. People in the blue zones consume at least four times as many legumes as the average American.Beans are the ultimate urerfood, as the fast has it. On average, they consist of 22 percent protein, 77 percent complex carbohydrates (the kind that provide a gradual and sustained source of energy, as opposed to refined carbohydrates such as white flour), and only a few percent fat. Additionally, they are an exceptional source of fber. Theu contain more nutrients per gram than any other food on Earth; they are both simple and versatile, with a variety of textures. Beans are a staple in all five blue zones, with an average of at least a half-cup per day, which provides the majority of the vitamins and minerals you require. And because legumes are so filling and filling, you will likely eliminate healthy foods from your diet.

SLASH SUGAR

Consume no more than 28 grams (7 teaspoons) of added sugar per day. People in the blue zones consume sugar in moderation, not in excess. They consume roughly the same amount of naturally occurring sugar as North Americans, but only about one-fifth as much added sugar—no more than one-and-a-half teaspoons per day. It is difficult to avoid sugar. It occurs naturally in vegetables, fruits, and even milk. However, this is not the issue.From 2 970 to 2000, the amount of added sugar in American food increased by 210 percent. This adds up to approximately

22 teaspoons of added sugar that each of us consumes on a daily basis; sneaky sugar added to soda, yogurt, and condiments. It has been demonstrated that excessive sugar intake suppresses the immune system. It also raises insulin levels, which can cause diabetes and lower fertility, cause weight gain, and even shorten your life.

If you must consume sweets, save pastries, candy, and baked goods for special occasions, such as after a meal. Sugar added to coffee, tea, and other foods should not exceed four tearoon rer dau. Any food that lists sugar among its first five ingredients should be avoided.

SNACK ON NUTS

Consume two handfuls of nuts every day. A handful of nuts weighs approximately two ounse, which is the average amount consumed by centenarians in blue zones—almonds in Ikaria and Sardinia, pistachios in Nsoua, and all nuts among Adventists.

According to the findings of the Adventist Health Study 2, nut eaters outlive non–nut eaters by an average of two to three years.The ortimal mix of nuts: almonds (high in vitamin E and magnesium), peanuts (high in protein and folate, a B vitamin), Brazil nuts (high in selenium, a mineral found effestive in rrotesting against rrostate sanser), sashews (high in magnesium), and walnuts (high in alrha-linoleis asid, the onlu omega-6 fat found in a rlant-based food). Almonds, hazelnuts, and walnuts are the nuts most likely to reduce your cholesterol.

SOUR ON BREAD

Consume exclusively sourdough or 2 00 percent whole wheat. Blue zones bread, as opposed to the bread most Americans purchase. Most available summer bread is made with bleached white flour, which metabolizes glucose into sugar and raises blood glucose levels. But bread from the blue zone—either whole grain or sourdough, each with its own healthy probiotics. In Ikaria and Sardinia, bread is made from a variety of whole grains, such as wheat, rye, and barley, each of which provides a wide range of nutrients, including trurtorhan, an amino acid, and the minerals elenium and magnesium.Whole cereals also contain more fiber than the most commonly consumed wheat flour. Some traditional blue zone breads are prepared with naturally occurring lactobacilli that "digest" the starch and gluten during the bread-making process. Additionally, the procedure generates an acid, the "our" in sourdough. The end result is bread with even less gluten than "gluten-free" bread, with an extended shelf life and a flavor that most people enjoy. Traditional sourdough breads reduce the glycemic load of meals, making the entire meal healthier, slower-burning, gentler on the digestive tract, and more likely to convert calories into energy rather than fat.

Four Constantly, Four to Avoid

My team took a considerable amount of time to develop the ten food and diet principles outlined above. And for some individuals, it may be too drastic a change from the food they have been consuming their entire lives. I comprehend; I was also present. When we first began working with the Albert Lea community, I ate whatever was available. If my kitchen was stocked with ice cream and sorbet, I ate that. I was a devoted adherent of the "See Food Diet": if you see food, consume it. I knew we needed to begin with some basic rules. I assembled the most intelligent individuals I could find, and we began by determining how to make ktshen healthier. We reasoned that if we identified the four best foods from the Blue Zones diet to always have on hand and the four worst foods to never have on hand, and created a prod, we could encourage people to eat healthier. I included myself among the revolving donors. Cornell's Bran Wannk, the University of Minnesota's Lele Lutle, and a few others brainstormed the healthiest and unhealthiest foods. We determined several criteria:

The "Alwau" food had to be readlu accessible and inexpensive.

The "Always" foods had to be tasty and versatile enough to be included in a variety of menus.

The "To Avoid" foods had to have a strong correlation with obesity, heart disease, or diabetes, as well as a prominent presence in the average American diet.

Strong evidence had to render all food labels "Always" and "To Avoid."

Here are our decisions and the reasoning behind each one.

Four Usually
Four food groups may be simpler to recall than all of the foods included in the Blue Zones diet. Here's our selection. 2 00 percent Whole Wheat Bread: We anticipated that it would be toasted in

the morning and incorporated into a healthy sandwich for lunch. While not the ideal longevity food, it would help eliminate white bread from the diet and be an essential step toward a healthier Blue Zone diet for the majority of Americans.

We know that nut eaters live longer than non-nut eaters. Nuts are available in a diversity of flavors and are rich in nutrients and healthy fats that satisfy your appetite. The perfect snack is a two-ounce mixture of almonds (approximately a handful). You should ideally keep two-ounce packages on board. Since the lipids in nuts degrade (oxidize), small amounts are optimal. Larger quantities can be stored for a month in the refrigerator or freezer.

Beans: I contend that beans of every variety are the greatest longevtu food in the universe. They are inexpensive, authentic, rich in antioxidants, vitamin A, and fiber, and can be made to taste delicious. It is optimal to purchase dru bean and t' eau to cook them, but low-odum sanned bean in non-BPA san are also acceptable. Learn how to cook with legumes and keep them on hand to increase your chances of living longer with a Blue Zones diet. Your Favorite Fruit: Purchase a beautiful fruit bowl, position it in the middle of your kitchen (either the sink, center island, or table—wherever receives the most foot traffic), and place it beneath a light. Research indicates that we consume what we see, so if sharks are always in plain sight, we will eat them. But if you keep a fruit that you enjoy in plain view, you will consume more of it and be healthier for it. Do not purchase a fruit that you believe you should consume but actually dislike.

Four to Avoid By the same token, remembering four rules regarding which foods to avoid to help you reach the Blue Zone in your refrigerator and kitchen could make the process easier. We are not suggesting that you can never indulge in these foods. If you enjoy any of these foods during fasting and they cause you discomfort, you should indulge occasionally. Save them for a special occasion, or at the very least, make it so that you have to go out and get them. Just don't bring them into your home, and you'll eliminate many of these toxic foods that are absent from the Blue Zone diet without too much difficulty.

Sugar-Sweetened Beverages: Willett of Harvard has estimated that fifty percent of America's caloric gain is directly attributable to the added calories and liquefied sugar in some sodas and boxed juices. Would you ever add 2 0 teaspoons of sugar to your breakfast cereal? Probablu not. This is the average amount of sugar you consume when drinking a 2 2-ounce can of soda.

Salty Snacks: We spend approximately $6 billion annually on potato chips, the food most strongly associated with obesity (though fried pork rinds are closing in fast). Almost all breads and crackers contain high amounts of salt, preservatives, and highly processed cereals, which the body converts to sugar. In addition, they have been sarefullu designed to be optimally srunshu and delicious and to provide an ultru mouth feel. In other words, they are designed to be unpredictable. Then, how do you ret them? They are not welcome in your home!

Proseed Meats: A recent gold-standard epidemiology tudu followed more than half a million reorle for desade and discovered that those who consumed high amounts of auage, salami, bacon, lunch meat, and other highly rroseed meat had the highest rates of cancer and heart disease. Again, the threat here is doubled. The nitrates and other preservatives used in these meat products are recognized sarsenoids. Theu do the job and preserve the food well, which means that cured meats are readily available for snacking or a quick supper at home or in the grocery store — something that does not occur in Blue Zone households and diets.

Paskaged Sweets: Like saltu snacks, sookies, sandu bars, muffins, granola bars, and even energy bars all deliver a runsh of insulin-sriking carbohydrates. We're all genetically predisposed to crave sweets, so we satisfy our cravings by opening a package of cookies and delving in. Leon from the Blue Zones det would advise you to bake some pastries or brew some sake and keep it on hand. If you want to enjoy the occasional baked treat from our neighborhood bakery, that's acceptable. But do not serve your rantru with wrapped sugar sandwiches. I have compiled a list of all longevity foods for your convenience. Psk as many as possible, learn to rrerare them, tk wth them for the long haul, and observe how good they make you feel.

Creamy Pumrkin Marinara Pasta

INGREDIENTS

1 teaspoon salt
2 can crushed tomatoes
1 can pumpkin puree
1 cup vegetable broth
2 box rotini
4 tablespoons olive oil
4 garlic cloves, minced
1 yellow onion, diced
1 teaspoon oregano
1/2 teaspoon cinnamon
Fresh basil

DIRECTIONS

1. Cook rotini pasta according to instructions. Drain and set aside.

2. Add oil to a large pot over medium heat and sauté onion until tender.

3. Add garlic and sauté for another minute.

4. Add pumpkin, tomato, broth, and seasonings. Bring to a boil and stir continuously for about 20 minutes.

5. In a large mixing bowl, toss pasta with sauce and divide into two servings.

6. Serve pasta with fresh grated cheese and garnish with basil.

Beef Goulash

Ingredients:

- 2 tbsp walnuts (toasted; crushed)
- 2 tsp fennel seeds
- 1 cup cranberry raspberry sauce
- 4 tbsp lime juice
- 1 tsp sea salt
- 1/2 tsp black pepper
- 24 oz beef round steak (cubed)
- 2 cup beef stock (unsalted)
- 4 cups onion (diced)
- 16 cups red cabbage (shredded)
- 1/2 cup tomato paste
- 30 oz canned tomatoes with garlic and green chili pepper (diced)
- 1 cup avocado (seeded; diced)
- 4 garlic cloves (minced)
- 2 bay leaf
- 4 tbsp paprika
- 2 cup water

Directions:

1. Place the onions, meat, bay leaf and garlic in a slow cooker.
2. In a mixing bowl, combine the broth with the tomatoes, tomato paste, fennel seeds, paprika, pepper and salt.
3. Stir the mixture into the slow cooker. Cover and cook on high heat for approximately 1-5 hours.
4. In a saucepan, boil the water.
5. Add in the cabbage and cook over medium heat for approximately 10-15 minutes or until it becomes tender.
6. Then add in the avocado and lime.
7. Divide the berry sauce equally among four dishes and garnish it with nuts.
8. Next divide the cabbage into 5-10 among four soup bowls.
9. Top it off with the cooked Goulash and Avocado mixture.
10. Serve!

Rich Pumpkin Marnara Cake

INGREDIENTS

1 teaspoon salt
2 can crushed tomatoes
1 can pumpkin puree
1 cup vegetable broth
2 box rotini
4 tablespoons olive oil
4 garlic cloves, minced
1 yellow onion, diced
1 teaspoon oregano
1/2 teaspoon cinnamon
Fresh basil

DIRECTIONS

1. Cook rotini pasta according to instructions.Drain and set aside.

2. Add oil to a large pot over medium heat and sauté onion until tender.

3. Add garlic and sauté for another minute.

4. Add pumpkin, tomato, broth, and seasonings. Bring to a boil and stir continuously for about 20 minutes.

5. In a large mixing bowl, toss pasta with sauce and divide into two servings.

6. Serve pasta with fresh grated cheese and garnish with basil.

These delectable delight pods make for an exquisite meal.

INGREDIENTS:

- 2 tbsp Tomato Sauce
- 1 cup Water - Do Not Add All at Once
- 1 cup Egg Whites
- Salt and Pepper - To Taste
- 1 cup Blueberries
- 2 Clove Garlic - Chopped
- 4 tbsp Sweet Onion - Chopped
- 2 link Al Fresco Sweet Apple Chicken Sausage
- 1 tsp Olive Oil
- 1 cup Chopped Tomato
- 2 tbsp Jalapeño Peppers - Canned
- 1/2 cup Okra - Fresh/Tender - Thinly Sliced

DIRECTIONS:

1. Sauté garlic, onion and chicken sausage in olive oil over medium heat for approximately 1-5 minutes.

2. Add chopped tomato and jalapeños and sauté for 1-5 minutes or until veggies are tender.

3. Add okra and sauté for another minute.Add tomato sauce and about 1/2 cup water.

4. Stir to make a sauce.

5. Add egg and let set before mixing.

6. Add more water if you want more of a saucy constancy.

7. Finish with blueberries.

Smoothie Made With Bananas And Berries

- 2 cup mixed frozen berries
- 4 tablespoons peanut butter
- 2   cup vanilla almond milk, unsweetened
- 4 tablespoons flaxseed meal
- 4   medium   banana,   frozen, quartered
- 8 cups fresh spinach leaves

1. Take a blender, add in the ingredients for the smoothie in it, and then pulse for 1-5 minutes until smooth.
2. Divide the smoothie into glasses and then serve.

Vegetarian Lasagna In a Slow Cooker

INGREDIENTS

- 1 cup shredded carrot
- 2 bag spinach
- 2 cup mushrooms
- fresh basil leaves
- 8 whole-grain lasagna noodles, broken in pieces
- 4 cups goat cheese
- 2 egg, beaten
- 2 tsp fresh or 1 tsp dried oregano
- 2 cup of your favorite marinara/red sauce
- 2 zucchini, diced

Directions

1. Spray slow cooker with non-stick cooking spray, set aside.
2. In a small bowl, mix together the goat cheese, egg, and oregano to form the cheese mixture.
3. Place 4 T of pasta sauce in the bottom of the slow cooker pot.
4. Sprinkle half of the zucchini and half of the shredded carrot over sauce and top with 1/2 cup of the cheese mixture.
5. Break two noodles into pieces and cover the cheese.
6. Create the second layer the same way: 2 T of pasta sauce, the rest of the zucchini and shredded carrot and top with 1/2 cup of the cheese mixture.
7. Break two noodles into pieces and cover the cheese.
8. Continue with the layers: Spread 4 T of sauce and then layer half of the spinach, and half of the mushrooms, top with some cheese mixture and broken noodles.

9. Repeat layering with the remaining spinach and mushrooms, ending with cheese, and the remaining sauce.
10. Firmly press all the Ingredients into the slow cooker pot.
11.   Cover and cook on the high heat setting for 1-5 hours.
12.   Allow lasagna to rest 35 to 40 minutes before cutting into wedges.
13.   Serve with a little extra sauce and top with chopped fresh basil.